C000131709

Easy Raw Soups
40+ Super-Easy, Nutrient-Rich
Raw Food Recipes
Bursting with Flavor

Green Reset Formula Book 3

Your guide to making rich and decadently creamy raw soups by using simple & inexpensive ingredients.

Joanna Slodownik

Copyright Joanna Slodownik, 2022. All rights reserved.
Disclaimer: This book is not a source of medical information. It provides information about the subject covered. The reader is encouraged to seek professional medical advice before taking action.

What's Inside

Why Raw & Living Soups?

SOUP IS THE ULTIMATE COMFORT FOOD, AND IT'S NICE TO HAVE IT hot, especially during cold wintertime, when you need something to warm you up.

So why make them raw?

Doesn't that defeat the purpose and negate the benefits?

Well, not really. You may be skeptical about making raw soups at first, but once you try them, you will appreciate how easy they are to prepare and how much energy they give you. You may have to get used to the taste of raw soups, when you try them for the first time you may not be convinced, but with each subsequent attempt they'll taste better, until finally you will fall in love with them.

Especially during the hot summer days, you'll find them refreshing, cooling, while also nourishing and satisfying. The great part is that you get the nutrients without getting the heavy feeling you may be used to after you eat. The vegetables are raw, full of vitamins and enzymes, which are no longer found in boiled soups.

Creamy tomato, cream of broccoli, cream of mushroom, etc., you get the picture. There are endless varieties of cream-based soups. Unfortunately, these soups are highly acidic, often putting you over the halfway mark for your recommended daily amount of sodium in one can. And yet, people enjoy these canned soups on a regular basis. Did I mention the amount of processed ingredients, preservatives, and unhealthy fats and oils that are in these soups?

What most people fail to realize is that healthy food can also be FAST FOOD, as in FIVE-MINUTE fast!

Seriously! (Unless you just eat vegetables and fruits whole or in salads, of course, but even then, it takes time to chop, bite and chew them well, while blended soups you can simply eat with a spoon or even drink.)

Here are some other benefits (and forgive me if I sound over-the-top here, but these are all benefits that I experienced and love):

* **Insane energy.** Eating raw foods provides an energy boost that must be experienced to be believed! You won't know this unless you try it for yourself. You know that feeling of being tired around 2 or 3 pm during the day? Eating mostly raw foods helps reduce that problem. When you do get tired, it doesn't last nearly as long, and a healthy snack or a bowl of raw soup will recharge you quickly.

* **Low in calories**, low in fat, low in sodium, and most are wheat-free and soy-free. These soups are cholesterol-free, dairy-free, lactose-free, and contain no chemical additives, or other unhealthful stuff.

* **High in nutrients.** Nourish your body, prevent disease, and improve your health. Boost immunity and help your body fight infections and diseases. Scientists agree, raw or cooked, just eat your veggies, and lots of them!

* **Eat as much as you want.** Yeah! This isn't really a health benefit, but it is pretty awesome, don't you think? You'll never get that uncomfortable full feeling when you're eating raw. The one when you have to unbutton the top button on your pants and just have to take a nap—you won't get that. You can eat as much as you want, and, while you will feel satisfied, you will not feel weighed down or tired. (*The only ingredients you need to be mindful of are cashews or other nuts, which are super healthy, but should be consumed in moderation.)

* **Less cleanup.** Simply put, there aren't many dishes to wash when you eat raw fruits and vegetables.

* **No packaging.** Eating raw means less packaging, which means less trash in your kitchen and landfills. Plus, more room in your cupboards. It's a win-win for you and the environment.

* **Better sleep and less sleep needed.** I notice I sleep better while eating more raw foods. But, most importantly, I wake up feeling less tired or groggy. On most days, I wake up full of energy.

* **Increased mental clarity.** Eating raw has helped me to focus better and be more emotionally in tune with others. This benefit is not easy to demonstrate; unlike a reduced waistline, it's difficult to show off or measure. It feels like a fog has lifted in my brain, and when I sometimes indulge in junk food, I notice how it makes me cranky and never fully satisfied. It's definitely easier to think clearly and focus for long periods when eating raw foods.

* **More regularity.** You should naturally have around two to three

bowel movements a day, with one being an absolute minimum. If you're going less than that, it probably means your intestines are clogged. A raw diet gives you more than enough fiber to keep you regular.

   * Impress your guests with a dish they didn't expect. The simple soups and blended salads in this book are super-easy to make, contain only a few simple ingredients, and yet have that look and taste that is sure to impress even the most discriminating guests. In fact, these soups are so tasty and elegant that you can serve them during holidays and other special occasions.

   * Serve chilled or warmed. You can serve these soups at room temperature or chilled (just add ice to your blender if you're pressed for time). Some of these soups can be warmed up, which will make them perfect comfort soup for the cold winter days.

   * Connection with the Earth. Eating food that's been freshly picked, minimally processed, and maybe even locally grown and in season, is better for the environment. Eating lots of processed foods—frozen or from a box—creates a gap and a disconnect from the planet that sustains us.

   * Kindness to other conscious beings on this planet. All recipes in this book are vegan, which means absolutely no animal ingredients.

   Seriously, don't you think it's just AMAZING!

   The thing I love about eating the raw foods is there's no cooking, no reheating, the food is easy to pack, it's fresh and colorful, and my hunger is satiated quickly. There's a minimal mess in making food, too, which is what I need.

   I need EASY. I need UNCOMPLICATED. I need FAST.

   I'm just one of those people who hate complicated recipes with a passion and find long preparation of meals exhausting—at least most of the time. Usually, I'm busy with other things and don't feel like using my brain cells to come up with stuff to have for dinner.

   So, are there any minuses? Well, some people may experience slight discomfort, which stems from two reasons. One is that if you're accustomed to eating heavy meals several times per day, then having a raw meal (even a big one) may not satisfy you for long. You'll be hungry much sooner than after a cooked meal—so you may still want to eat some cooked food, including not-so-healthy-stuff, except you'll probably eat much less of it. Second, you may experience discomfort in your gut. Both are minor disadvantages, and they should not deter you from adding more raw plant foods to your diet!

It should be noted that I don't recommend you go 100% raw to see the benefits of eating this way. Any increase in raw foods in your diet will give you noticeable, immediate results.

This book isn't about becoming a raw-foodist; it's about ADDING MORE WHOLE PLANT FOODS to your diet in the easiest possible and delicious way.

In fact, you shouldn't change your diet too quickly. Small steps are best, so start slowly, especially if you have any serious health issues. If you are mostly healthy, you can be more daring, but always, always LISTEN TO YOUR BODY.

While slight discomfort is okay, pay attention to any foods that give you adverse reactions. For some, it may be cruciferous veggies, for others it may be raw garlic or onions, or other.

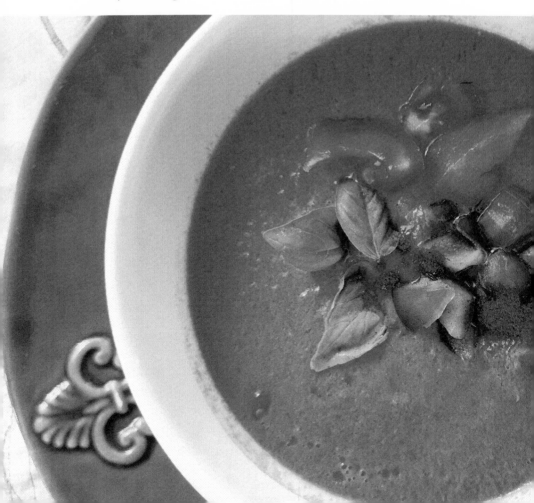

Tips for Full Flavored Raw Soups

1.   Choose high quality ingredients

Get the freshest, highest quality raw vegetables, greens, fruits & herbs you can find. Finding ingredients that are locally grown, in season, and organic is ideal, but not always possible. Vegetables, including leafy greens, offer the soup chef an infinite number of culinary possibilities. Not only are they an essential part of a healthy diet, they also have countless nutritional benefits.

2. Add liquid

Adding liquid is optional in these soups. Most of the soups are more like thick stews and can totally be made without adding any liquid (in which case you have to make sure you add plenty of watery ingredients, such as tomatoes). With that said, if you prefer a thinner soup, **add some water, unsweetened non-dairy milk, or freshly made juice**. It's important that you don't dilute the soup too much, so be sparing with your liquid at first.

3. Add creaminess to your soup

Blending the soup on high speeds will make it creamy, but **adding ripe avocado, cashews, almonds, or cashew cream** (see the recipe at the end of the Raw Soup Recipes section) will take that creaminess to a whole new level. Also, check out **the emulsification method** described in the Traditional Gazpacho Recipe. It takes a bit more time, and contains some oil, but it's totally decadent and worth to try.

4. Deepen the flavor

If you use fresh, ripe fruits and vegetables and add fresh herbs, then the soup will be delicious on its own. However, if you are used to very salty, spicy, and fatty foods, your taste buds may need some time to adjust. Learn to use herbs and spices as the main seasoning, and limit the use of salt. Experiment by adding your favorite fresh and dried herbs and spices, such as chili powder, cilantro, cinnamon, coriander, cumin, curry powder, dill, fennel seed, garlic, ginger, marjoram, mustard, nutmeg, oregano, paprika, parsley, red pepper/cayenne, rosemary, sage, tarragon, thyme, and turmeric. Add an acid (lemon juice, apple or wine vinegar) to soup to perk it up. Vinegar adds a bite to soup, and there are many varieties available, including wine vinegar, balsamic, sherry vinegar, and fruit-flavored vinegars.

Chili sauce, tabasco, sriracha, ginger, lemon juice, soy sauce, tamari, miso, and pesto are just some of the many flavorings that can add depth to soups.

5. Garnish like a pro

You've used great ingredients. You've cooked and salted them properly. How to make the most of it all before it hits the table? Add a bit of something fresh right at the end. Fresh herbs are my favorite, with dill, parsley, and cilantro being the ones I use the most. Top with freshly squeezed citrus juice, a dollop or two of cashew cream, and a handful of diced fruits and veggies. Sprinkle with flaked almonds or other nuts and seeds. Roast them first for a few minutes on a hot frying pan for a deeper flavor.

6. Serve with bread, cooked beans, potatoes, or grains

If you are concerned that a bowl of raw soup will leave you hungry, serve it with a side of whole grains such as barley, couscous, millet, quinoa, cooked beans, cooked potatoes, pasta, rice noodles, tofu, or a slice of bread. You may not need to even cook; just check your pantry or refrigerator, as leftovers are great for this purpose.

7. Serve them warm or chilled

Serve the soup the way that is convenient and appeals to you the most—warm, chilled or at room temperature. Simply blending the soup for a longer time will warm it up, or heat it gently on the stove. For a chilled soup, refrigerate it for an hour or more, or if pressed for time, just add ice instead of water.

8. Take your time

For some people, raw soups may not be love at first spoonful. Especially, if you don't eat many raw vegetables and salads, you may need to get used to the taste and consistency, but with each subsequent attempt your taste buds will adjust, until finally you will fall in love with them. Give yourself time to adjust and experiment and make it fun.

If you find yourself struggling with making these soups appeal to you (or your loved ones), try a recipe with avocado or the **Traditional Gazpacho Recipe**. It's a bit more involved, plus it contains some oil and bread, but it's almost a guaranteed hit.

Smoothies, Soups, Stews, Juices— Oh, My!

Sometimes the difference between them can be blurry, especially since many recipes use similar ingredients. So, what's the difference between a raw soup that contains, say, celery and apple, from an apple-celery smoothie?

For me, it all comes down to spices and how it is served. I like to add some salt and pepper to my soups, plus spices that are usually associated with savory dishes, such as curry, cumin, etc. I also serve soup in soup bowls and eat with a spoon, while I drink my smoothies from a glass.

The difference between soup and stew can be even fuzzier. Stew has usually more "grainy" texture, although I do like to top my creamy soups with lots of diced ingredients, so there you go!

To add to this confusion, even though the title says "Raw Soups," it doesn't mean that all the ingredients have to be raw. Adding some leftover grains, for example, will make the whole meal a lot more filling.

The whole idea is to have fun. Our taste buds may have to adjust to these new flavors, but once they do, you may find yourself experimenting in your kitchen, mixing and blending ingredients you'd never imagine could be eaten together or raw. Once you come up with a great combination, you'll be dancing in your kitchen with your spoon and plunger, as I sometimes do, wondering why it took you so long to discover all these wonderful flavors.

Essential Tools for Great Soups

These soups only take about 5-10 minutes to make, with the most complex recipes requiring up to an hour of prep time start to finish, including cleaning. It doesn't get much easier and healthier than that!

1. Blender

A blender is all you need to make these soups. You may use any blender you have, but if you're shopping for a blender, I recommend a high-power blender, like a Vitamix or Blendtec. It will allow you to make delicious soups, sauces, cashew cream, almond milk, and other recipes—it's an incredibly versatile kitchen appliance. Vitamix comes with a tamper to push foods down that comes in handy when making thick soups and stews. In my opinion, a tamper is essential for many raw food recipes. Without it, the recipes may take longer to prepare, and you may have to use higher speeds. These blenders are not cheap, but consider it an investment in your health. Vitamix comes with a 7- year warranty and is so well-made it will probably last you a lifetime. To save money, find a used one or buy a refurbished unit. With all that said, any blender—even hand-held mixer—will do the job.

2. Juicer

Optional, but nice to have. After my blender, my juicer is my second favorite kitchen appliance. Blended soups can be quite thick, so straining some pulp or adding some fresh juice to your soup can thin it a bit, without losing the flavor. If you don't have a blender, juicing some ingredients and chopping the rest can be an excellent method to make raw soups. You may add some of the pulp back into the mix to thicken the soup.

3. Sharp knife, chopping board & peeler

Adding diced fruits, veggies, and herbs will add delicious texture to your soup.

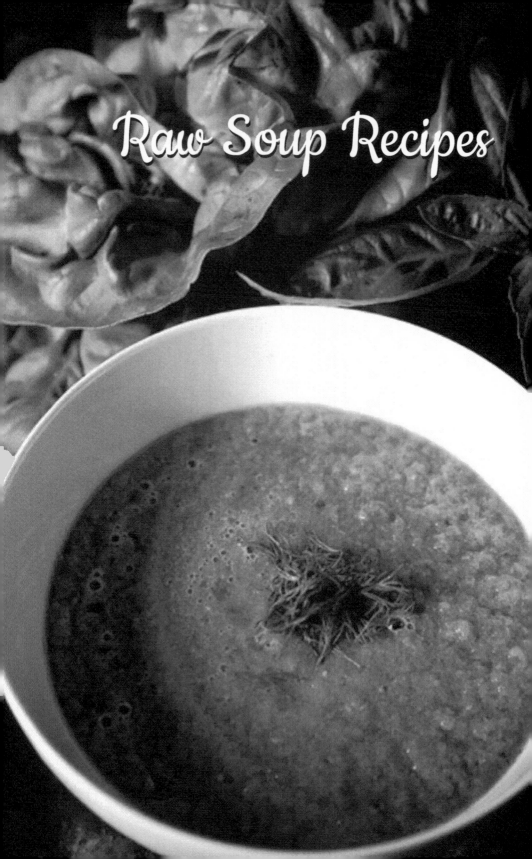

Raw Soup Recipes

Broccoli Cucumber Soup

THIS RAW BROCCOLI-CUCUMBER SOUP IS FULL OF NUTRIENTS, YET VERY LOW IN CALORIES. It strengthens the immune system; plus broccoli (and other cruciferous vegetables) contains potent anti-cancer and anti-aging compounds. It only takes a few minutes to prepare this soup, so there is no excuse not to make it!

INGREDIENTS
   1/3 cup broccoli florets
   1 large cucumber, peeled and cut into pieces
   1 teaspoon of lime juice
   Sea salt and pepper to taste

METHOD
   Blend until smooth (depending on your blender, it may take from 10 to 30 seconds or even longer) to get broccoli nice and creamy. Serve chilled with a squeeze of lime juice and a few sprinkles of dill or dried mint.

VARIATIONS
   Make this soup with Brussels sprouts instead of broccoli.
   Add 1/2 of avocado for a more creamy soup.

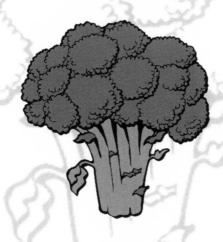

Broccoli Avocado Soup

Many raw soups can be made with avocado as the base. Just blend everything with cilantro or mint; and then serve it with arugula, cherry tomatoes, or strawberries. So, here is a creamier (and higher calorie) take on broccoli soup. Total preparation time: 5 minutes.

INGREDIENTS

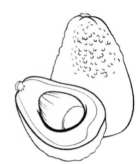

2 cups almond or cashew milk
2 cups broccoli florets
1/2 stalk celery, chopped
1 avocado, de-seeded
1 tablespoon onion
1 clove garlic
1/2 teaspoon cumin
Salt and pepper to taste

METHOD

Blend until smooth (depending on your blender, it may take from 10 to 30 seconds or even longer) to get all ingredients nice and creamy. Serve immediately, or refrigerate for a couple of hours to meld the flavors. Bring back to warm (as in baby-bottle warm) before serving.

Green Reset Energy Soup

INGREDIENTS

3 leaves of Swiss chard or other mild leafy greens
1 stalk celery
1 large avocado
½ bunch fresh parsley
1 lemon, juiced
1-2 cups water

METHOD

Blend all ingredients until smooth. Adjust thickness by adding water. Season to taste with salt and pepper. Stir into soup: grated carrot, grated cauliflower, some raw corn kennels, and/or sprouts.

Raw Gazpacho

GAZPACHO IS CONSUMED THROUGHOUT SPAIN AND PORTUGAL. This is a simplified version of this all-time favorite. For the Traditional Gazpacho Method, go to page 52. It's best to make this soup a day ahead to allow the flavors to meld together.

INGREDIENTS

6 vine-ripened tomatoes, peeled, seeded, and chopped
1 stalk celery, chopped
1/8 small red onion
1 small garlic clove, minced
1/2 cucumber, peeled and sliced
1/2 red bell pepper, cored and seeded
2-3 tablespoons fresh basil leaves, parsley, or cilantro
1 tablespoon freshly squeezed lemon or lime juice
2 teaspoons balsamic vinegar
1-2 cups vegetable or tomato juice or water (to desired consistency)
Salt and freshly ground pepper to taste

METHOD

Blend all tomatoes, celery, onion, and garlic at high speed until smooth; add the rest of the ingredients and blend at low speed until the soup reaches desired consistency—do not over-process (the soup should have a bite to it). Add juice or water, if desired, to achieve the desired thickness. It should not be too thin.

Cover and refrigerate for one hour or more, allowing flavors to combine. The longer gazpacho sits, the more the flavors develop. Mix well and serve chilled. Garnish with chopped vegetables, herbs, and/or croutons, if desired.

Season to taste. Experiment with adding your favorite spices, including salt, pepper, thyme, oregano, marjoram, basil, tarragon, and celery seed. For even more kick, add a piece of jalapeno pepper, Tabasco sauce, Worcestershire sauce, etc. Gazpacho can be refrigerated overnight.

Peach Gazpacho

SWEET PEACHES REPLACE TRADITIONAL TOMATOES in this savory fruit version of gazpacho.

INGREDIENTS

6 ripe peaches (about 2 ½ pounds), peeled, halved, pitted, and cut into chunks
½ medium cucumber, peeled, seeded, and cut into chunks
1 small garlic clove, minced
½ to ¾ cup water
1 teaspoon apple cider vinegar or champagne vinegar, or to taste
2 tablespoons fresh flat-leaf parsley or cilantro, chopped
Salt and freshly ground pepper to taste

FOR GARNISH

Finely chopped red bell pepper and avocado

METHOD

Pulse ½ cup water, the peaches, cucumber, garlic, vinegar, oil, ½ teaspoon salt, and ¼ teaspoon pepper in a food processor until coarsely pureed. Thin with more water if desired. Refrigerate for at least 2 hours.

Season with vinegar, salt, and pepper. Stir in herbs. Garnish with bell pepper and avocado. Drizzle with oil and sprinkle with salt. Gazpacho can be refrigerated overnight.

Sweet Apple-Dill-Avocado

INGREDIENTS

4 stalks celery
1 bunch dill
2 apples
1 avocado
1 lemon
1-2 cups water

METHOD

Blend all ingredients until very smooth.

Creamy Celery & Garlic Soup

The cashews create the creamy base for this raw soup, which is surprisingly filling. It has a refreshing aspect to it, which is not characteristic of creamy soups made with dairy. The celery has a lot to do with that, that's excellent for your health. A blender is required, and you can blend the soup for about 3-5 minutes on high to naturally warm it up. That's the perfect hack to add a little warmth to your soup!

INGREDIENTS

1 cup celery, roughly chopped
1 tablespoon raw cashews
1/2 garlic clove, minced
1/2 cup filtered water
Salt and pepper to taste
1/2 cup celery, finely chopped and reserved

METHOD

Add all the ingredients, except the 1/2 cup of chopped celery for garnish, to a blender and blend on high until smooth.

Leave the soup blending for a few minutes to warm it up.

Pour the soup into a bow and top with the chopped celery. Season with optional sea salt and pepper and enjoy. Serves: 1.

Celery & Pear Soup

INGREDIENTS

1 cup celery, roughly chopped
1 cup zucchini
1 pear, roughly chopped
1 cup water
Salt and pepper to taste

FOR GARNISH

Fresh herbs, such as dill or cilantro, chopped
Diced pear

METHOD

Blend all ingredients until smooth. Adjust to taste and desired thickness. Serve chilled in bowls garnished with fresh herbs.

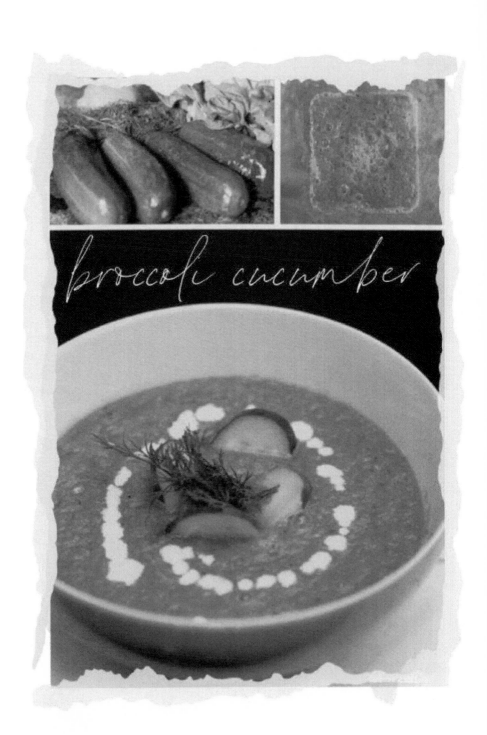

broccoli cucumber

Avocado-Cucumber Soup

INGREDIENTS

2 ripe avocados, halved, pitted, peeled, and diced
4 cucumbers, peeled, seeded, and chopped
½ jalapeno pepper, seeded and finely diced (optional)
½ cup chopped fresh cilantro, plus a few springs for garnish
4 tablespoons fresh lime or lemon juice
1 clove garlic
½ cup of water or plant milk
Salt and pepper to taste

FOR GARNISH

½ cucumber, thinly sliced
1 radish, julienned
½ red bell pepper, cut into strips
½ cup fresh corn kernels

METHOD

Put the avocados, cucumbers, jalapeno pepper, cilantro, lime juice, lemon juice, water, and a dash of salt, if using, in a blender and process until smooth. Taste and adjust the seasonings if needed. Cover and refrigerate until chilled, about one hour, or up to 3 hours. Ladle the soup into bowls and garnish each portion with radish, bell pepper, corn, and cilantro.

VARIATIONS

Substitute cilantro with chopped fresh dill for tasty cucumber-dill soup. Add 1 cup chopped spinach or lettuce. Garnish with cashew sour cream. To make cashew sour cream, squeeze some lemon juice into thick cashew cream (see the Cashew Cream Recipe).

Thai Green Soup

INGREDIENTS

2 cucumbers
5 kale leaves
1 large avocado
1 lime, juiced
2 cloves of garlic
½ inch fresh turmeric root or ½ teaspoon of turmeric powder
½ inch fresh gingerroot or ¼ teaspoon dried ginger powder
1-2 cups water

METHOD

Put all ingredients into your blender and whizz until smooth. Taste and adjust the seasoning. Pour into individual bowls. Garnish with cilantro and serve!

Red Pepper Soup

INGREDIENTS

1 red pepper
1 avocado
2 cups of water
1/4 cup mixed cilantro & parsley
Pinch of oregano
Salt and pepper to taste

METHOD

Blend all ingredients until very smooth. Taste and adjust the seasoning. Pour into bowls. Enjoy!

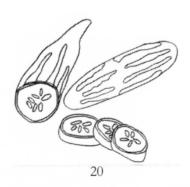

Raw Cream of Kale

KALE IS WELL KNOWN FOR ITS ANTI-INFLAMMATORY AND ANTI-CANCER properties. It is high in beta-carotene, vitamin K, vitamin C, and calcium, among other goodies. I'm a big fan of kale—I love putting it in my green smoothies and juices. This is another excellent way to have it.

INGREDIENTS

3 cups of almond milk
6 big kale leaves, stems removed
1/2 clove of garlic
1/8 onion
1 lemon, juiced (or more)
3 tablespoons of nutritional yeast flakes
Salt and pepper to taste

METHOD

Soak 1 cup almonds for a few hours or overnight. Blend almonds with 3 cups water on high until very smooth, about one minute. For very smooth milk, strain the pulp using cheesecloth (optionally).

Blend all ingredients for 4-5 minutes in the Vitamix. Blending it for so long will warm up the soup. Alternatively, you may blend your soup and then warm it up a little on the stove until you see steam rising out of the top. Pour the soup into individual bowls and garnish with fresh herbs, pumpkin seeds, and/or sliced mushrooms.

The nutritional yeast flakes are nice to have at hand in your kitchen. It will give the soup a cheesy flavor without using dairy. Plus, it's a source of vitamin B12. Season to taste with salt and pepper. Add a few whole peppercorns into the blender or about 1/8 of a teaspoon of freshly ground black pepper.

VARIATIONS

For a thicker soup, reduce the almond milk by half a cup. To make it cheesier, add more yeast flakes. If you want the soup a little tangier, add more lemon juice. Taste it until you're happy with it and enjoy!

Sequoia's Calcium Soup

This soup requires more ingredients than the previous recipes, but results in a deeper and more interesting flavor. It's a great raw soup for kids and a fantastic way to introduce vital heavy minerals and calcium into everyone's diet. (Recipe by David Wolfe.)

Ingredients

10 kale leaves
1 handful of parsley
2 cloves of garlic
1/3 of a red onion
2 lemons
1 avocado
1 tomato
2 yellow bell peppers
1 handful of dulse strips or Spirulina flakes
1/2 teaspoon sea salt
1 tablespoon of unpasteurized miso
3 tablespoons oil
20 pumpkin seeds

Method

Shave the outer skin of the lemons, leaving the white pith intact. While blending all the ingredients, add some water to reach a soupy consistency that you like.

Livefood Soup with Cilantro & Lemon

INGREDIENTS

1 cucumber with peel
1 red pepper
2 stalks celery
1 small tomato
1/2 beet
1 carrot
1 whole lemon, yellow peel removed
1-inch ginger root
3 cloves garlic
1/2 large red onion
1 bunch cilantro
1/2 cup fresh ground sesame seed
2 heaping tablespoons unpasteurized miso
1/4 cup olive oil
1/4 tsp. cayenne, to taste
Water, about 2 1/2 cups

METHOD

Grind the sesame seed in your coffee grinder for a few seconds to a moist meal. Chop veggies down and assemble all ingredients into your blender.

Depending on how much power your blender has, you may have to shred harder vegetables. This soup keeps well for a day or two in a sealed container in the refrigerator, so make some extra tonight for the next day's lunch. (Recipe by Annie & David Jubb)

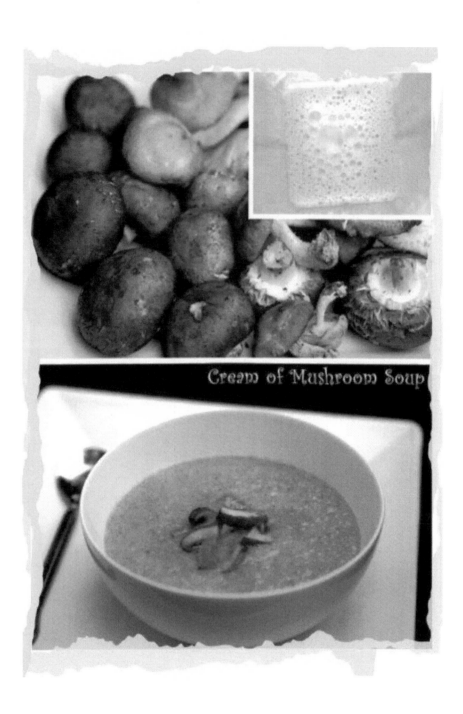

Cream of Mushroom Soup

Raw Cream of Mushroom Soup

INGREDIENTS

8 ounces of mushrooms, any kind you like
1 cup almonds (pre-soaked)
3 cups of water
1 garlic clove (optional)
a few whole peppercorns
sea salt to taste
a few fennel leaves or fresh dill for garnish

METHOD

To make almond milk, soak the almonds for a few hours or overnight. Blend almonds with water on high until very smooth, about one minute. Optionally, you may strain the pulp for smoother milk, but I usually skip this step when making a soup.

To make the soup, put the mushrooms in the blender container, pour enough almond milk to cover the mushrooms (2-3 cups), and blend on high until smooth. Taste and adjust the seasonings and liquid to desired consistency. Garnish it with a few fennel leaves or fresh dill.

VARIATIONS

Serve this soup raw or cooked, cold, or warm.

To make this soup steamy hot using your high-power blender (such as Vitamix), run it for 3-4 minutes on the highest settings. Alternatively, you may also heat it on the stove.

Substitute almonds with cashews to make cashew cream or use store-bought, unsweetened almond milk.

Raw Butternut Squash Soup

This is an exquisite soup to impress your guests. It's also very satisfying, especially with the pumpkin seeds.

INGREDIENTS

3 cups butternut squash
2 cups almond milk, or more to desired consistency
1/2 clove garlic
1 small chunk onion
1/8 teaspoon of cumin
1/8 teaspoon of curry powder
A few whole peppercorns
2 teaspoons of agave syrup, maple syrup, or another sweetener
A dash of cinnamon
Salt to taste
Raw pumpkin seeds for garnish, optional

METHOD

Blend until smooth in your blender.

To make this soup steamy hot using your high-power blender (such as Vitamix), run your blender for 3-4 minutes on high. Alternatively, you may also heat it on the stove. Taste and adjust the seasonings and liquid to desired consistency.

VARIATIONS:

Make this with sweet potatoes, squash or pumpkin.
Substitute almond milk with cashew cream.

Corn & Cashew Chowder

A perfect way to enjoy corn when it's in season!

INGREDIENTS

3 cups of raw sweet corn kernels plus 1/2 cup for garnish (about 4 large ears)
2 cups of water
1/2 cup raw cashews
1/2 clove garlic
Sea salt to taste
2 teaspoons chopped cilantro for garnish
Freshly ground pepper for garnish

METHOD

Blend everything but the garnishes until silky smooth. Pour into bowls, garnish with some fresh corn, a dash of black pepper, sprinkle a little on, and some chopped cilantro. The corn chowder can be refrigerated overnight.

Easy-Cheesy Tomato Soup

Here is another variation on the tomato soup theme. Nutritional yeast flakes add a creamy, cheesy flavor to this soup.

INGREDIENTS

6 medium-sized tomatoes
1/4 cup of raw cashews
1/4 cup of nutritional yeast flakes
1 teaspoon of sea salt

METHOD

Blend all ingredients until smooth and creamy. Tomatoes contain a lot of water, so start without adding any additional liquid, and adjust thickness as needed (you may not need any). To make this into a steamy, hot soup, let the blender run about 4 minutes.

Garnish with some fresh black pepper, basil, or broccoli florets.

Easiest Ever Creamy Tomato Soup

You only need two ingredients, tomatoes, and cashews, for this soup, so make sure the tomatoes are ripe and flavorful. The recipe will also work with quality canned tomatoes.

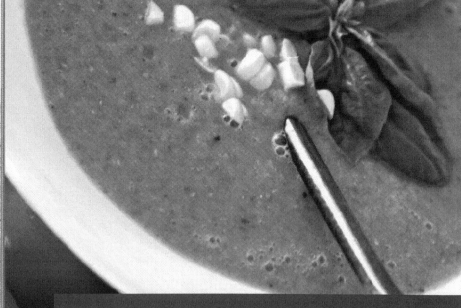

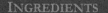

INGREDIENTS

One quart chunked tomatoes
1/4 cup raw cashews
Salt or garlic salt to taste or a blend
of the two (optional)

METHOD

Put tomatoes and cashews in the blender container and blend on high until very smooth. You may toss in a few basil leaves into the mix for a basil-flavored soup. I find I don't need seasoning with this soup, but you may like to add a little salt. Be careful when seasoning; remember, you can't take it out! For a warm soup, continue blending on high for a few minutes, or heat on the stovetop. Pour into soup bowls and enjoy!

Raw Tomato Basil Soup

INGREDIENTS

    4-5 tomatoes (cherry tomatoes are delicious in this recipe)
    4 sun-dried tomato slices
    1 cup fresh basil leaves, plus extra for garnish
    1 avocado
    1 celery stalk
    1-2 cloves garlic
    1/8 yellow onion
    1/4 cup fresh lemon or lime juice
    Dash of cayenne
    Salt and pepper to taste

METHOD

Place all ingredients in a high-speed blender or food processor and blend until almost smooth, or until desired consistency is reached. If using a regular blender, you may need to add extra water to help the mixture blend. Replace the basil with an equal amount of fresh cilantro, dill, mint, oregano, or tarragon—or experiment and find a tasty combination of herbs.

VARIATION

    4-5 medium tomatoes (cherry tomatoes are great for this recipe)
    2 cups loosely packed basil leaves, plus extra for garnish
    2 cups raw cashews, soaked
    1 tablespoon agave syrup, 4 soaked, pitted, and chopped dates or another sweetener (optional)
    1 cup of water
    1/4 yellow onion, finely chopped

Place cashews and water in a blender and blend until creamy. Add basil, tomatoes, and onion. Season with salt and pepper. You may use heated water to make the soup warm. You may also blend all ingredients on high in a high-powered blender for a minute or two until it's warmed and creamy. If using a Vitamix, the longer you blend in the first step, the warmer your soup will be. You may also heat your soup in a pot on the stovetop.

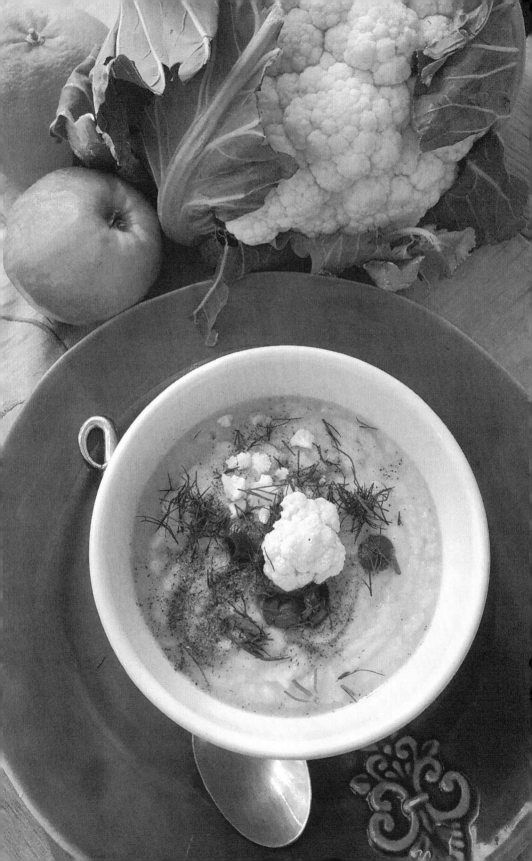

Raw Cream of Cauliflower Soup

When people hear about a raw cauliflower recipe, they express consternation about eating this cruciferous gem in the raw soup or smoothie. But there's no reason to be afraid. With its super mild taste and pleasantly crunchy texture, raw cauliflower is a highly palatable treat! The trick is, of course, to prepare it in a pleasing way. And nothing could be more pleasing than this rich and creamy recipe, which elevates cauliflower and autumn spices to a new level of perfection. It's very reminiscent of regular cream of cauliflower soup, but uses pine nuts in place of dairy.

INGREDIENTS

½ head (4 heaping cups) chopped cauliflower
½ cup pine nuts
2 tbsp olive oil
4 large dates, soaked and pitted
1 tbsp mellow white miso
1 tbsp lemon juice
1 cup water
½ tsp nutmeg
½ tsp celery seed
1/8 cup chopped onion or ¼ tsp onion powder (optional)
¼ tsp cinnamon
1/2 tsp salt
Salt and pepper to taste

METHOD

Blend all ingredients in a blender or food processor till well combined. Sprinkle with a touch of nutmeg, and enjoy! (Serves 2-3)

Apple Cauliflower Soup

INGREDIENTS

1 tablespoon of cashews (you may blend them first with water on highest setting until smooth and creamy)

1/2 large cauliflower

1 cup water

2 apples, peeled

1/2 grapefruit or lemon, juiced

Salt and pepper to taste

METHOD

Place all ingredients except salt and pepper in a high-speed blender. Blend until completely smooth. Sprinkle with salt and pepper to taste.

Top with marinated onions (see recipe below), apple slices, chopped fresh dill, or olives, if desired.

Serve chilled.

VARIATIONS

Instead of cashews, you may add 1 tablespoon olive oil (optionally, or skip the fats completely)

1 tablespoon apple cider vinegar Instead of olive, add

Instead of apple cider vinegar, use juice of grapefruit or lemon

MARINATED ONIONS

1 sweet onion, thinly sliced

2 tablespoons nama shoyu (tamari or soy sauce will also work)

1 tablespoon agave or other liquid sweetener

2 tablespoons olive oil

Mix together nama shoyu* (or regular tamari or soy sauce), agave and olive oil. Pour over sliced onions in a glass container with cover. Marinate onions for 2-3 hours, redistributing marinade a couple of times during marination. (*In Japanese, nama means raw, or unpasteurized, and shoyu means soy sauce; so, nama shoyu is a raw, unpasteurized Japanese-style soy sauce.)

Raw Curry Cauliflower Soup

Here's another variation on the raw cauliflower theme. (I really love raw cauliflower!) When you're not in the mood to cook, but still want to enjoy a healthy and hearty meal, you can whip up this soup in minutes. It's perfect for any time of the year. Serve warm or cool and be satisfied with some of the healthiest nutrients, spices and herbs.

INGREDIENTS
1/3 cup raw cashews
1 cup fresh young Thai coconut water & coconut
2 tsp extra virgin olive oil
1 medium shallot
1 medium head cauliflower, cut into 1-inch pieces
2 tbsp curry powder
1 tsp ground turmeric
1 tsp ground cumin
5 drops stevia (optional and to taste)
1/4 tsp ground cinnamon
1/4 cup chopped fresh cilantro
Salt and pepper to taste

GARNISH
Cubed avocado
Apple chopped into sticks
Trail mix, pepitas, coconut, raisins, assorted nuts & sunflower seeds for crunch (be creative!)

METHOD
Blend all ingredients except garnish in a high-speed blender until slightly warm, about 4–5 minutes. Garnish with preferred toppings and enjoy! (Serves 4-6.)

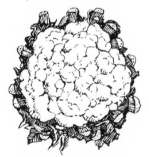

Raw Thai Carrot Soup

INGREDIENTS

    1 cup carrot
    ½ cup red pepper
    ½ cup water
    1 tablespoon lime juice
    2 teaspoons soy sauce
    1 teaspoon ginger
    1 garlic clove
    1 teaspoon lemongrass minced
    1 teaspoon scallion or onion
    Tai red chili pepper to taste

METHOD

Put all ingredients into your blender and whizz until smooth. Taste and adjust the seasoning. Pour into individual bowls. Garnish with cilantro and serve!

Carrot Pepper Soup

INGREDIENTS

    half an onion
    4 carrots
    1 red bell pepper
    2 cloves of garlic
    Italian herbs, oregano, dried ginger, cayenne pepper
    chopped nuts and basil

METHOD

Blend all the vegetables to the consistency of cream. Sprinkle with nuts and basil. Season generously with spices to your taste (the soup is better when it is spicy).

Carrot Avocado Soup

INGREDIENTS

4 medium carrots, peeled and chopped
2 ribs celery, chopped
1 large avocado
1/4 medium onion, chopped
1 clove garlic, pressed
Pinch of salt, or to taste
1 1/2 cups water or coconut water

FOR GARNISH

1/2 medium tomato, finely chopped
1 green onion, sliced

METHOD

Coarsely chop all the ingredients to make blending easier. In a blender, add everything but the tomato and scallion and teaspoon olive oil. Blend until very smooth. In some mixers, the soup will warm up a bit as it processes. Garnish with chopped tomatoes and scallions, and drizzle with a bit of olive oil.

TIP

If you grow your carrots or buy them with green tops, why not add some of those greens to the soup? Just chop them and add to the blender.

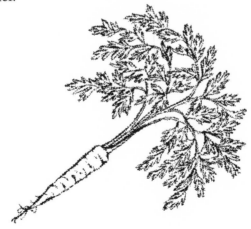

Carrot Coriander Soup

The fresh herbs and coriander (seeds of the cilantro plant) bring a fresh, earthy taste, and the avocado adds creaminess and texture. You can even use bottled carrot juice, or stop at a juice bar and get some fresh juice to make your life easier!

INGREDIENTS

2 cups fresh carrot juice

2 teaspoons of minced fresh ginger (add more for a little more warmth)

1 medium avocado, cut into chunks, pit removed

1/2 cup fresh leaves of cilantro

1/4 cup fresh leaves of parsley

2 teaspoons coriander seed (freshly ground is best)

2 tablespoons tamari sauce (optional) Pinch of salt, or to taste

FOR GARNISH

2 green onions, outer skin removed and finely sliced

Freshly crushed coriander seed or white and black sesame seeds

METHOD

Blend the carrot juice, ginger, and avocado at medium-high speed until smooth. Remove cilantro and parsley leaves from the main stems. Add in de-stemmed herbs, coriander seeds, and tamari. Pulse at medium speed until well mixed but with small pieces of herbs still visible. Season with a pinch of sea salt, if desired. Sprinkle green onions on top. Serve chilled. Garnish with crushed coriander seed or white and black sesame seeds as available.

Celeriac & Apple Soup

You may be skeptical about using celeriac (or celery root) in a raw soup, but trust me on this one: celeriac flavor compliments the tart green apple in this soup in the most delightful way!

INGREDIENTS
4 cups celeriac, peeled and roughly chopped
1 cup chopped green, tart apple, plus 1/2 cup for garnish
1/2 cup raw cashews
1 cup of water
1/4 cup lemon juice
Salt and freshly ground black pepper to taste

FOR GARNISH
1/4 cup minced chives
fresh dill

METHOD
Blend the celeriac and green apple until smooth. Add the cashews, water, and lemon juice and blend thoroughly. Season with salt and pepper to taste.

If not serving right away, store it in the refrigerator in a covered container. Bring it back to room temperature before serving (blending it again can help speed this process along as the movement increases the temperature), taste again, and adjust seasoning. Garnish with the diced apple, chives, or dill.

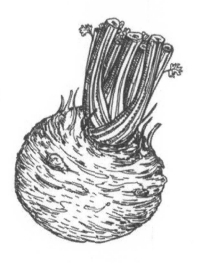

Creamy Zucchini & Celeriac Soup

This creamy zucchini and celeriac soup is a great winter dish. Delicious served in warm bowls.

INGREDIENTS

¼ white onion, roughly chopped
½ celeriac, roughly chopped
2 zucchinis, chopped
1 stalk celery, chopped
1 avocado, roughly chopped
2 tablespoons fresh dill or 1 tablespoon dried dill
2 tablespoons lemon juice
1 cup filtered water or coconut water, or more
1 teaspoon garlic powder
Salt and fresh pepper to taste

FOR GARNISH

Fresh herbs, chopped

METHOD

Combine all the ingredients in a high-speed blender and blend with 1 cup of filtered water. Adjust to taste and desired thickness. Serve in a soup bowl garnished with a sprinkle of fresh herbs. If it's wintertime, you may warm the soup up on the stove, simply place in a pot and stir gently over low heat. Remove just before the first wisp of steam rises. Serve in warm bowls.

Beet Soup (Borscht)

This soup is not only pretty and tasty, but incredibly healthy. Beets are both highly cleansing and loaded with nutrients: the agent that gives them their incredible color is a potent cancer-fighting compound. It is slightly sweet, but the sweetness is cut by adding apple cider vinegar, the creaminess of the avocado, and the spring of dill.

Ingredients

1 cup beet juice
1 cup carrot juice
½ cup apple juice
¼ tsp salt and a sprinkle of pepper
1 tsp apple cider vinegar (more to taste)
1 small beet, chopped (or half of a large one)
1/3 medium avocado (so ¼ of an extra-large one and ½ of a small one)
½ grated carrot
¼ grated beet
¼ chopped avocado
Spring of dill

Method

Blend all the ingredients in a blender, stopping to adjust saltiness and sweetness. You can let your soup sit overnight to allow the flavors to blend. It tastes great warm or hot, so heat it on the stove, if you like. Pour into bowls and garnish with the chopped vegetables. If you don't have a juicer, make the soup using a blender. If it's too thick, strain some of the pulp with a sieve.

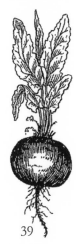

Creamy Beet Soup

BEETS ARE FULL OF LOTS OF GOOD VITAMINS, MINERALS AND NUTRIENTS so you know you're eating something good here! A beautiful color with amazing flavors, you can never go wrong with beets.

INGREDIENTS

2 to 3 medium size peeled beets
1/4 cup cashews (this will give it a more creamy flavor, you can omit it and just add more water)
Juice of 1/2 lemon
Salt and pepper to taste 1–2 cloves of garlic
Some chopped Jalapeño (optional)
Water—start with about 3/4 cup and add more depending on how thick or thin you like your soup

METHOD

Put all ingredients together into a blender and blend.
Blend until smooth.

FOR GARNISH

Fresh herbs - parsley, cilantro, and green onion.

Sweet Chilled Cherry Soup

A bowl of fresh fruit soup is a great way to begin or end a meal during the summer.

INGREDIENTS

1 1/2 cup cold almond milk
1 cup frozen cherries
2 tablespoons fresh lemon juice
a pinch of salt
chopped dates for garnish, optional
dried, shredded coconut, optional

METHOD

Blend cherries with almond milk and lemon juice. Garnish with chopped dates and shredded coconut flakes. Serve chilled.

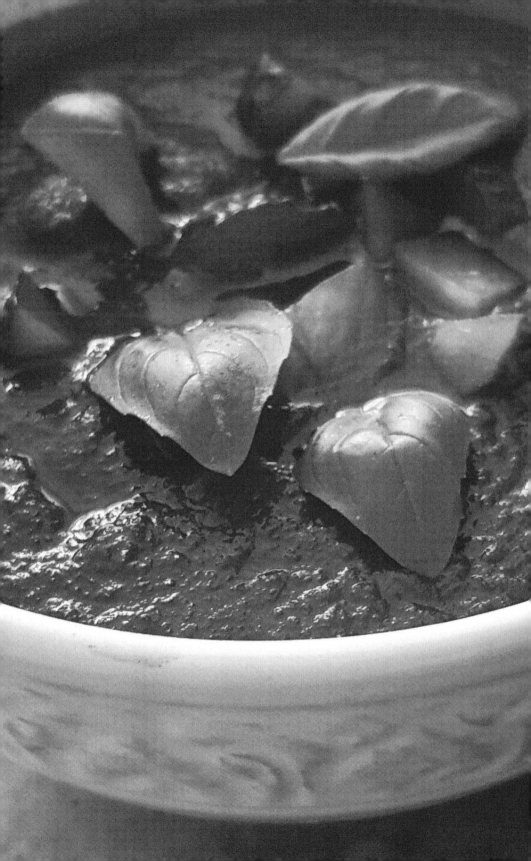

Ginger-Peach Soup
with Cashew Cream

THIS SOUP IS BEST MADE WHEN PEACHES ARE RIPE AND PLENTIFUL, but use frozen peaches that have been defrosted if you are making this out of season. For a decadent flourish, make some extra cashew cream and swirl a spoonful into each portion of soup.

INGREDIENTS

  1/2 cup raw cashews
  1 cup water, or more, as needed
  1 1/2 pounds ripe peaches, peeled, pitted, and sliced
  2 teaspoons fresh ginger peeled and grated (optional)
  1/2 cup fresh orange juice, apple juice, or 1/4 cup frozen orange juice concentrate
  1 tablespoon fresh lemon juice
  Agave, sugar, or another sweetener, if needed to taste
  Fresh mint sprigs for garnish
  Chopped peach pieces for garnish

METHOD

  Place the cashews, water, peach slices, ginger, orange juice, and lemon juice in a blender and process until very smooth. Add a little more water if the soup is too thick.

  Taste and adjust the seasonings, adding a little sugar, if needed, for sweetness. Pour into a container with a tight-fitting lid and refrigerate until well chilled. Serve cold, garnished with the mint sprigs and chopped cashews.

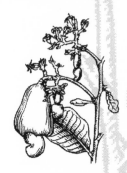

Cashew Cream Recipe

MANY OF THE RECIPES IN THIS BOOK USE CASHEWS. Here is how to make some cashew cream in advance and simply add it to the soup.

Let me tell you—cashew cream is beyond amazing. Even though it's exactly a low-fat, low-calorie, or cheap ingredient, a little goes a long way, and it's definitely worth it when you want to make your soup a special occasion.

Many chefs know this secret and are using cashews in their dishes. Since I tried them, I love them so much, I've been using cashews in various recipes, not just soups. They are a fabulous and versatile ingredient.

Be sure to use raw cashews to avoid the distinctive flavor of roasted cashews. Unlike roasted cashews, raw cashews have little flavor of their own. Because of the fat content, cashew cream reduces in a pan even faster than heavy cream. This recipe is for about 2 1/4 cups thick cream or 3 1/2 cups regular cream.

Take 2 cups whole raw cashews (whole are better than pieces, which are often dry) and rinse them under cold water. Cashews don't really need to be soaked before use, but if you like, simply put them in a bowl and add cold water to cover them, and refrigerate overnight. (I usually skip this step.)

Place cashews in a blender with enough water to cover them by 1 inch. Blend on high until very smooth. If you're not using a high-speed blender (such as a Vitamix, which creates an ultra-smooth cream), strain the cashew cream through a fine-mesh sieve. Or use a dry blender or coffee grinder and grind into a paste, then mix in the water and add to the recipe.

To make thick cashew cream, simply use less water so that the cashews are barely covered by the liquid.

To make sour cashew cream, add a dash of lemon juice or vinegar.

In the raw-food world, cashew cream is often used in soups and desserts. Once prepared, store it for up to 3 days in the refrigerator or freeze for up to 6 months (although once defrosted, it can get lumpy, so you may need to give it a spin in the blender before using).

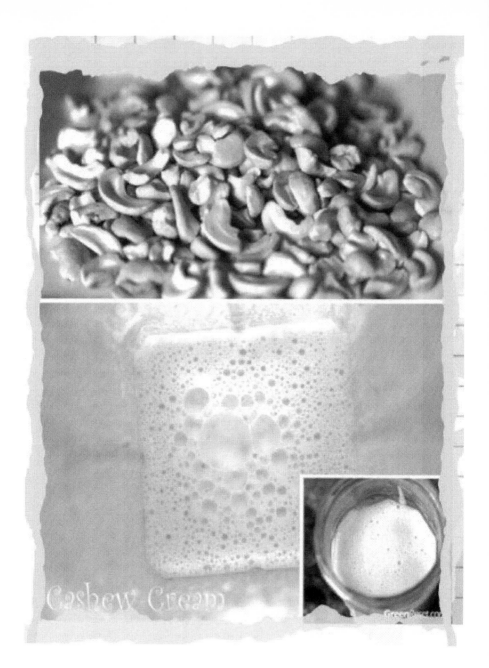

Cashew Cream

Note: Cashews are excellent sources of healthy fats, including both monounsaturated and polyunsaturated varieties. Although they aren't the best source of protein, they do contain a small amount per serving. One thing to be mindful of in regards to cashews, or any nut for that matter, is that you don't want to eat them in excess. Nuts typically contain a lot of calories per serving, consume them sparingly. I know how easy it is to just keep snacking on them without realizing how much you're consuming, so just be mindful of that.

Thick Raw Veggie Stew Recipes

IN THIS CHAPTER, I WANT YOU TO START EXPERIMENTING and creating your own thick veggie stews with ingredients that you find in your farmer's market or garden, based on a few basic principles and recipes below. Blended stews are similar to soups, but thicker because they're made without adding liquid. They are made of primarily juicy vegetables and greens and blended at lower speeds and shorter times than smoothies, with no additional water.

They have thicker consistency, crunchy texture, and can be eaten from a bowl like a soup or stew. The best ingredients for blended salads include tomatoes, cucumbers, celery, peppers, and zucchini, with only delicate greens added, such as spinach or lettuce. The reason not to add hard and bitter greens such as kale is that you are only blending the mixture to a consistency of thick salsa or stew—and these ingredients would make it unpalatable.

Be sure to add lots of herbs, such as basil, dill, parsley, cilantro, and others, for even more flavorful dishes. Sprouts are also terrific to add to the blend or just sprinkle on top. If you don't have fresh herbs, dried herbs are fine. Experiment with other condiments, such as curry powder, hot sauce, onion, or garlic, to create a greater variety of tastes.

Even though a stew is a savory dish, adding some sweetness is highly recommended. I like to add some sweet fruit: a piece of pear, apple, a few strawberries, or grapes, but you may choose to add a little bit of agave, a dash of stevia or another sweetener, or a few dates, soaked, pitted and chopped.

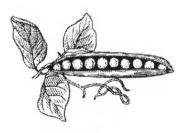

Basic Raw Veggie Stew Recipe

THIS IS A BASIC RECIPE TO GET YOU STARTED. Once you get the idea of how to make these, you can create your own variations easily. There are practically unlimited combinations, so you could make a different one every day for the rest of your life. Use the freshest ingredients you can find for the best flavor and nutrition.

KEY POINTS TO REMEMBER:

1. Add ingredients in the order stated in the recipe to your blender, starting with the watery ingredients FIRST to create a base for the soup.

2. Always blend at the lowest speed that gets the job done, don't over-process. Blend at the slowest possible speed and least amount of time possible to get the job done. During this entire process, my Vitamix usually never gets beyond the speed of 7 or 8. Start slowly and increase speed if needed.

3. No need to pulverize it and bring it to a froth. Just get it down to a liquid base. Nice to have some texture in there.

4. Add sweetener to kick the flavor to the next level.

5. If you don't own a blender with a tamper, you may use a celery stalk or carrot to push the ingredients down into the blender blades.

START WITH MAKING THE BASE FOR THE STEW:

2-3 ripe tomatoes halved or quartered (save one half for the topping)
1 large or medium cucumber peeled or not peeled (1/2 English or seedless cucumber) You may only use half of the cucumber for this part. The other half can be used as a topping (optional)
1 large stalk celery (optional)
Blend these ingredients until smooth in your blender. This is your base.

THEN ADD:

2 scallions chopped into quarters or smaller
2 or more teaspoons agave syrup, maple syrup, or another sweetener

1 small red Thai Chile pepper (optional or add a jalapeno or your other favorite hot peppers to taste.)
Blend until the above mixture is liquefied

THEN ADD:

5 ounces of spinach or other greens (use less in a regular household blender, about 3 ounces)

Add greens gradually, not all at once. Remember to blend at the lowest speed that gets the job done. By adding the greens gradually, you can use a slower speed, which will put less strain on your blender's motor. Note: for regular or low power blenders, you might have to add the spinach in smaller amounts to get the job done without burning out your motor.

Last, but not least—

ADD YOUR TOPPINGS:

Chop the tomato and cucumber that you saved. You can also cube some extra sweet red, yellow, or orange pepper, zucchini, and celery. Add on top and or mix in with a spoon and enjoy.

VARIATIONS:

You may vary your base, as well as greens and toppings to your heart's content. For example, you may only use tomatoes, tomatoes, and cucumber, or you may also toss in sweet red, orange, or yellow peppers. A heartier substitute for cucumber is organic zucchini. Zucchini is also a fantastic topping to use, as it almost tastes like potatoes.

NEXT, ADD IN YOUR SEASONINGS:

There are unlimited combinations, but don't add too many of these per stew. Remember, simple is usually much better. These are choices, and you may wish to use these by themselves or to combine with other herbs or spices:

basil
cilantro
dill
Thai basil
sage
tarragon
parsley
mint
chives

scallions
green onions
cumin
other fresh herbs and dried spices of your choosing
yeast flakes
dulse flakes
soaked kelp or dulse leaves
curry powder
onion flakes
garlic
hot pepper, jalapeno, etc.
salt and pepper

ADD SWEETENER:

Although we're not making green smoothies here, adding some sweetener takes this dish to a whole new level. Try adding:

soaked dates

sweet fruit, such as pear or apple

raw agave nectar, maple syrup, or another sweetener

(Dates can be soaked overnight or longer to be soft. Or chop them up a bit before soaking, so you wont' have to soak as long.)

GREENS:

spinach, romaine, Boston lettuce, iceberg lettuce, mixed or baby greens

Add about 5 ounces total. That's not including the herbs, which are greens as well, and can be a substantial portion of the mixture.

You can add fewer greens if you wish and make it more of a soup or a thinner consistency.

Or just add more tomatoes and or cucumber to make it thinner.

TOPPINGS:

Just chop up any or all of these—tomato, zucchini, cucumber, celery, tomatillo, apple, sweet peppers, and even raw okra. The more colors, the more beautiful it looks. This step is optional. You don't have to chop any toppings up if you're short on time.

So, now let us try a few variations.

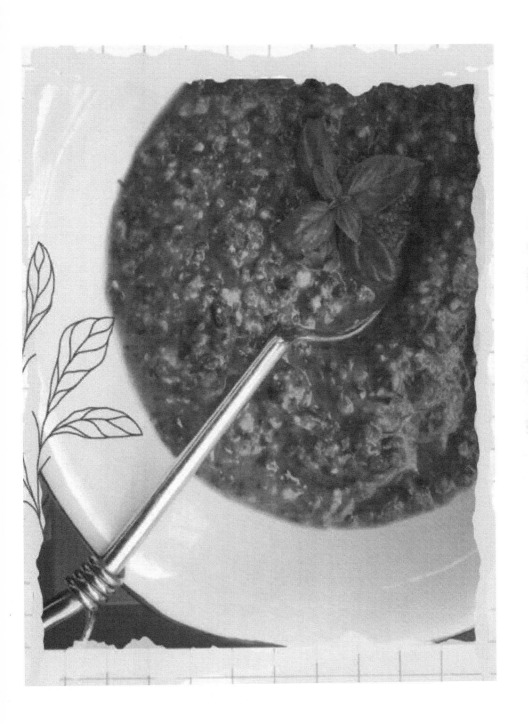

Thick Zucchini Stew

INGREDIENTS

2 tomatoes
2 medium green zucchinis
2 scallions
curry powder
4 teaspoons of raw agave nectar or another sweetener
jalapeno or other hot pepper (optional)
6-8 large stalks celery
Add the ingredients below in the order stated and liquefy in your blender.

START WITH

2 tomatoes halved or quartered (leave half for the topping)
2 medium peeled green zucchini (leave a piece for the topping)

NEXT, ADD

2 scallions chopped into quarters or smaller
1 tablespoon curry powder (to taste)
4 or more teaspoons of raw agave nectar or another sweetener
2 slices jalapeno pepper (optional or add your other favorite hot peppers to taste.)
Blend until the above mixture liquefies.

NEXT, ADD

6-8 large stalks celery
Pour liquid into a bowl. Chop or cube and mix in the rest green zucchini. Also, mix in 6 stalks of chopped celery.

TOPPINGS

Chop or cube the remaining tomato. You can also chop in extra sweet red, yellow, or orange pepper and celery. Sprinkle a handful of chopped cilantro and a handful of dulse flakes.
Enjoy!

Italian Stew

INGREDIENTS

2 tomatoes
1 medium to large cucumber or ½ English or seedless cucumber
1 large stalk celery
2 scallions
fresh basil (more or less to taste)
fresh oregano (can substitute dried oregano)
a dash of raw agave nectar or another sweetener
jalapeno or other hot pepper
5 oz spinach

OPTIONAL TOPPINGS

a handful of sweet bell pepper, diced
1 chopped celery stalk

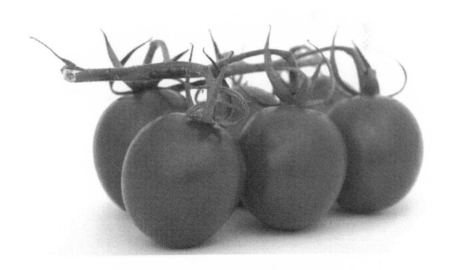

Tex-Mex Stew

- 2 tomatoes
- 1 medium to large cucumber
- 1 large stalk celery
- 2 scallions fresh cilantro
- a dash of raw agave nectar or another sweetener
- jalapeno or other hot pepper
- 5 oz spinach or other tender leafy greens

OPTIONAL TOPPINGS

a handful diced sweet bell pepper, 1 chopped celery stalk, 1 diced avocado, chopped tomatillo, pico de gallo (chopped tomato, tomatillo, onion, jalapeno pepper, cilantro, and lemon juice)

Sweet & Spicy Thai Stew

INGREDIENTS
- 2 tomatoes
- 2 medium green zucchinis
- 2 scallions
- fresh ginger
- Thai basil
- fresh cilantro
- a dash of raw agave nectar or another sweetener
- jalapeno or hot pepper
- 9 large stalks of celery
- bell pepper
- dulse flakes

Blend all ingredients until the mixture liquefies. Enjoy!

Traditional Gazpacho Method

I'm very fond of gazpacho and other Spanish coolers, but if I order them in restaurants, but I am often disappointed when I get a watery and bland cocktail, tasting like vinegar. The real gazpacho has a distinct vegetable flavor, and it's velvety with lots of chunks of fresh cucumbers, peppers, or tomatoes. That's why Ishare with you a recipe and a handful of tips on how to make a really decadent tomato cooler, taking inspiration from the tricks used in two types of Spanish cold soups, gazpacho and salmorejo.

What's most important in a good Spanish gazpacho?

* **Good quality of ingredients, in this case, tomatoes:** this is a cliché, but it's worth repeating. Hard, sour, poor-quality tomatoes will make the soup taste just like that. It pays to find ripe, fragrant tomatoes, especially raspberry or buffalo hearts. In the case of the latter, instead of 5 pieces, 2 or 3 will suffice; after all, they can be really huge.

* **Bread:** it was bread and oil that formed the basis of the first Spanish gazpacho, such as cojondongo or salmorejo. The memory of this ingredient is not only of historical value; the addition of bread thickens the soup, adding fluffiness and density. If you avoid gluten, use gluten-free bread (I know, it's pretty obvious) or possibly 1/4 cup of almonds or cashews, which should be soaked in boiling water for 30 minutes. Almonds, like bread, thicken the soup and add delicious volume, as is wonderfully demonstrated in a cooler called ajo blanco.

* **Salting the vegetables in advance:** instead of simply throwing the vegetables in the blender, blending and adding salt as you go, it's much better to salt them and let them sit on the counter for about half an hour. This small change makes a huge difference - it makes the vegetables soften and let the juice out right away, which makes the gazpacho easier to blend into a silky texture and, most importantly, it won't dilute after it's done.

* **Emulsification:** often the oil is simply poured on top of the soup, but the key to perfect gazpacho to the emulsification process. It may sound complicated, but it's really nothing difficult. Emulsification is the process of permanently combining two non-combining substances, in this case vegetable juice and oil. The same way a vinaigrette sauce or mayonnaise is made. To make gazpacho emulsify, all you need to do is first blend the

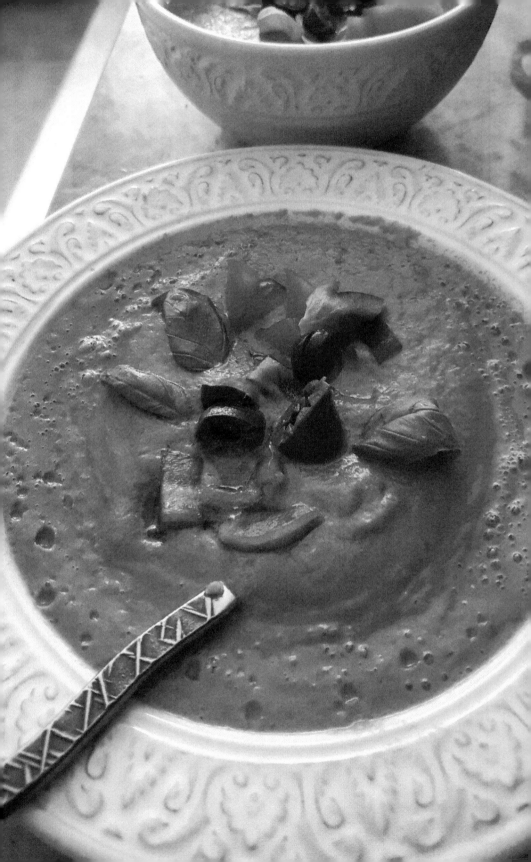

vegetables for a while with a fair amount of vinegar, and then pour in the oil very slowly. This will make the texture much smoother and velvety. This process takes a little longer, but it's definitely worth the wait!

Traditional Gazpacho Recipe

Preparation time: 15 minutes + 30 minutes waiting time

INGREDIENTS (FOR 3 - 4 SERVINGS)
5 tomatoes, preferably raspberry
1 red bell bell pepper
2 ground cucumbers
½ red onion
1 teaspoon salt
3 slices of baguette or soft bread (can be stale)
2 ½ tablespoons apple cider vinegar or wine vinegar
¼ - ½ teaspoon agave syrup
a pinch of chili, optional
¼ cup olive oil
To serve: chopped cucumber, bell pepper and black pepper, optionally, olives, cherry tomatoes, or other veggies

METHOD
Peel the cucumbers, then roughly dice them with all the other veggies, sprinkle with salt, add the baguette broken into pieces and put them in a large bowl. Mix and set aside for 30 minutes, and preferably for 1-2 hours.

Strain the vegetables in a sieve over a bowl, collecting the juice in a bowl. Put the drained vegetables in the blender, add vinegar, agave syrup and chili and blend everything thoroughly. Add the vegetable juice and blend another minute at high speed, then slowly pour in the olive oil.

Finally, season to taste with salt and pepper, if desired, and serve with lots of chopped vegetables.

TIPS
The soup can, of course, be blended with a hand blender. You can also add 1 clove of garlic.
The bread can be stale dry. To be honest, I always use just such.

Gazpacho with Smoked Paprika

This is another gazpacho that combines traditional salmorejo with gazpacho andaluz. This combination is simply heavenly. From the andaluz gazpacho I took the proportions, the balance of flavor and the crunchy vegetables on top; and from the salmorejo I took the technique of thickening with bread and emulsifying with oil. And then there's the all-important trick that applies to any kind of gazpacho, which is to salt and set the vegetables aside. This is what allows the vegetables to be left in their skins, so the cooler has that deep, intense flavor; but at the same time it is smooth, because the vegetables can soften properly thanks to the salt.

If you are not sure whether such a procedure makes sense, I have a suggestion - try doing it this way at least once, and you will see for yourself that all the previous gazpacho will no longer mean anything to you. Preparation time: 15 minutes + 30 minutes of waiting.

INGREDIENTS (FOR 4 - 5 SERVINGS)
   5 tomatoes, preferably raspberry
   2 red peppers
   2 ground cucumbers
   1 red onion
   1 teaspoon smoked paprika
   1 teaspoon salt
   3 slices of baguette or soft bread
   2 ½ tsp. apple cider vinegar or wine vinegar
   2 Tbsp. ajvar, optional
   ¼ -½ teaspoon agave syrup or sweetener of choice
   ¼ teaspoon chili flakes
   ¼ cup olive oil
   To serve: chopped cucumber, chopped bell peppers and chilies

METHOD
   Peel the cucumbers and, along with all the other vegetables, cut them into coarse cubes, add salt, smoked paprika, a baguette broken into pieces and put them in a large bowl. Mix together and leave on the counter for at least 30 minutes, and preferably for 1 - 2 hours.

   Strain the vegetables in a sieve over a bowl, saving the juice from the vegetables in the bowl. Put the drained vegetables in the blender cup, add vinegar, agave syrup, chili and optional ajvar and blend everything thoroughly. Add the vegetable juice and blend another minute on high speed, then slowly pour in the olive oil.

Season to taste with salt and more vinegar if needed, and serve with chopped cucumbers and peppers and an extra pinch of chili.

White Gazpacho (Ajo Blanco)

White gazpacho or ajo blanco, is a delicious cold soup originating from the Andalusian region of Spain.

When summer comes around, cold soups start popping up on restaurant menus everywhere. Spanish red gazpacho is the epitome of cold soups. This recipe however, is for the lesser known gazpacho- white gazpacho or ajo blanco, meaning white garlic. White gazpacho is actually the original gazpacho. It originated in the Andalusian region of Spain before tomatoes were introduced to the country. Andalusia was occupied by the Moors for hundreds of years in the Middle Ages. Their Arabic culture influenced the food of that region.

White gazpacho uses inexpensive ingredients like olive oil, garlic, stale bread and almonds, which grow abundantly in that region of Spain. Almonds and olive oil provide heart healthy unsaturated fats. Almonds additionally provide protein and fiber as well as several other nutrients that have beneficial effects on heart health. Cucumbers and grapes are packed with water to keep you hydrated.

Traditionally made with a mortar and pestle, the base of white gazpacho consists of blanched almonds and garlic that are mashed into a paste. You want to make sure to use blanched almonds which have the skins removed since the skin adds a slightly bitter flavor. It also changes the color of the soup.

Stale bread (soaked in water to soften it) and olive oil are then added to form an emulsion. Although traditional white gazpacho uses a large amount of olive oil, you can cut down on the amount without sacrificing the taste or texture of the soup.

Cucumbers, grapes and a shallot are then added to provide fresh, vibrant flavor as well as a touch of sweetness to mellow out the garlic.

A splash of Spanish sherry vinegar adds the right amount of acid to round out the dish.

Here's the last thing to know about ajo blanco: Even after you've followed the recipe, you've blended it and chilled it and given it time to settle into itself, if you try it just like that...you may not be impressed. Try to hold your judgment until you've eaten the finished, plated soup, because ajo blanco isn't ajo blanco without its fruit garnish.

That's true of a lot of soups—the garnish elevates it from an everyday experience to a special affair. Ajo blanco just isn't a fully realized dish until it's studded with juicy, sweet-tart bites—usually fresh grapes, or other fruit, like melon.

Once you try ajo blanco in that state, it'll go right to the top of your cold-summer-soup list.

INGREDIENTS

2.5 ounces cubed white bread (about 2 cups) from a baguette, Italian loaf or sliced bread (crust cut off)

1 ½ cups cold water, divided use

⅓ cup whole, blanched almonds

1 clove garlic

2 tablespoons chopped shallot

2 cups diced, peeled English cucumber (about 1 large cucumber)

¾ cup green grapes

2 tablespoons extra virgin olive oil

3 ½ teaspoons sherry vinegar

1 teaspoon salt

Chives or scallions for garnish (optional)

METHOD

Put the bread cubes in a bowl and pour ½ cup water on top to soften them. Put the almonds and garlic in a blender and puree until finely ground. Add the shallot, cucumber, grapes, oil, vinegar, salt and softened bread to the blender along with the remaining 1 cup water. Puree until smooth. Taste and adjust salt as needed. Add more water to the soup as needed to achieve desired consistency.

After blending, you'll want to put the soup in the fridge, giving it enough time for the flavors to meld and develop. Serve in bowls or glasses and garnish with sliced grapes, almonds and chives or scallions if desired.

VARIATIONS

Get creative and try different varieties of gazpacho like watermelon or peach.

Coconut Cucumber Kohlrabi Cooler

In Eastern Europe, people are used to kefir- or buttermilk-based coolers, meanwhile, on the cooler map of the world you can find a variety of inspiring vegan recipes. Among the most famous is certainly Spanish gazpacho, a cold soup made of tomatoes and bread, but equally refreshing is Andalusian white gazpacho, called ajo blanco. It's prepared a little differently in each city, but the main ingredients are almonds, garlic and grapes, which are mashed with water and finally turned into an emulsion by adding olive oil.

This coconut kohlrabi cooler is crisp, spicy and disarmingly creamy. Coolers of all countries, run for the coconut milk and kohlrabi!
Preparation time: 10 minutes

INGREDIENTS (FOR 2 - 3 SERVINGS)
1 can of coconut milk (400 ml)
1 cup of plant milk, such as rice milk
4 - 6 tablespoons of lemon juice
½ clove of garlic
Salt and pepper to taste
1 kohlrabi
1 cucumber
2 radishes
To serve: chives, mint, freshly ground pepper

METHOD
Blend both milks, lemon juice, garlic and a generous pinch of salt in a blender to a smooth liquid.

Cut the vegetables into small, even cubes, add to the liquid and mix with a spoon. Put in the refrigerator for an hour, after which time serve with chives, mint and fresh pepper. It tastes best the next day, when the vegetables have released their juice. Great as a lunch for work.

TIPS
You don't even have to use a blender to make this soup. Just grate the garlic and simply mix all the liquid ingredients in a bowl.

From Ignorance to Awareness

The Best Foods for Optimal Health & Weight

THE FOLLOWING RECOMMENDATIONS ARE BASED ON THE 'EAT TO LIVE' PROGRAM: The Revolutionary Formula for Fast and Sustained Weight Loss by Dr. Joel Fuhrman, which is a book that I cannot recommend enough. I feel it should be required reading in school and college (together with other books by this author.) You should definitely read those books yourself, but in the meantime, here is the gist of what doctor Fuhrman recommends:

UNLIMITED (eat as much as you want):

Fresh, raw greens, vegetables, and fruits (unlimited). 60-80% of what you eat should be RAW (or lightly cooked) plant food. Make huge salads as main dishes or side dishes to your cooked soups, or prepare **raw soups** (see the recipes at the end of the book for Live Cucumber Soup, Gazpacho, and other). Drink green smoothies and green juices.

Steamed/lightly cooked green vegetables (unlimited, goal one pound daily). Spinach, kale, collard greens, Swiss chard, escarole, dandelion, beet greens, all lettuces, herbs, etc.

Non-starchy vegetables (unlimited). Peppers, onions, tomatoes, eggplants, etc.

Mushrooms, cooked, and raw (unlimited). Mushrooms are probably one of the most underrated, underappreciated ingredients out there—and yet they provide fantastic health benefits, including stimulating the immune system, helping to fight infections and cancer. Plus, they are excellent for weight loss, as they contain about 80 to 90% water and are very low in calories (only 100 cal/oz). They have very little sodium and fat, and 8-10% of the dry weight is fiber. Add mushrooms to soups, salads, and sandwiches. I include several recipes for mushroom soups, but toss in a few mushrooms to any soup to enhance its flavor and nutrition.

Legumes: beans, bean sprouts, peas, lentils, soybeans (including tofu), and other (unlimited, minimum 1 cup daily in total of these.) High in fiber and antioxidants, beans aren't just good for the waistline; they may aid in disease prevention, too. They are also high in calcium and iron, plus they are a fantastic source of protein. Dry beans that have been soaked and cooked are an excellent source of nutrients and a great ingredient to add to any soup. A great idea is to prepare enough beans to use in different dishes throughout the week.

The nice thing is—you may have as much of these foods as you like—in soups, salads, side dishes, and as snacks!

LIMITED (no more than one serving if trying to lose weight):

Cooked starchy vegetables OR cooked grains—Maximum 1 cup per day. These include butternut or acorn squash, corn, sweet potato, cooked carrots, brown rice, whole-grain bread, whole-grain cereals. Avoid highly processed breads and cereals as much as possible.

Raw nuts and seeds (1 oz. or 28.5 grams a day) or 2 ounces avocado. Nuts and seeds are great and very healthy but are high in fat and calories, so don't go overboard with them. The recipes you find in this book use cashew nuts—but only in small amounts to enhance the flavor and texture. Raw nuts and seeds can be added to salads to add some crunchiness. They are especially nutritious when pre-soaked or sprouted. They are optional for overweight persons who follow a weight loss plan because of high fat and calorie content.

Ground flaxseed (1 tablespoon per day)

Non-dairy milk, such as soymilk, low-sugar preferred—maximum 1 cup a day, optional.

Dried fruits, such as dried dates, raisins, etc. minimal amounts, less than one serving (doctor Fuhrman puts dried foods on the off-limits list, so use them sparingly only as a treat).

OFF-LIMITS:

Dairy products
Animal products
Soft drinks, fruit juice
Salt, sugar

People who still have difficulty losing weight may also eliminate starchy vegetables, grains, nuts and seeds, dried fruits, and stick to limited amounts of low-sugar fruits.

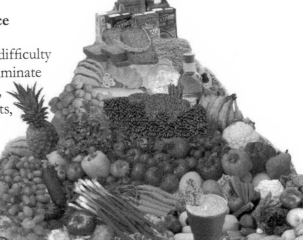

Be Mindful of Fat
(Even Olive Oil) in Your Soup

ALTHOUGH OUR BODIES REQUIRE FAT TO FUNCTION, THE BEST SOURCES to get healthy fats are whole plant foods, such as raw nuts, seeds, leafy greens, avocados, beans, and other unprocessed ingredients. Adding refined fats is entirely unnecessary and can add a lot of calories to an otherwise low-calorie meal. Americans consume far too much fat, an estimated 60 grams of added fat in the form of oils, which is over 500 empty calories per day. Refined or extracted oils, including olive oil, are rich in calories and low in nutrients.

There are a lot of calories in just a little bit of oil. This may surprise you, but ounce for ounce, olive oil is one of the most fattening, calorically dense foods on the planet. It packs even more calories per pound than butter (butter 3,200 calories; olive oil 4,200). The bottom line is that oil will add fat to our waistlines, heightening the risk of disease, including diabetes and heart attacks.

Fat contains about 9 calories per gram, while protein and carbohydrates contain approximately 4 calories per gram. So when you eat high-carbohydrate foods, such as vegetables and beans, you can eat more food and still keep your caloric intake relatively low. It is usually the small amount of added refined fat or oils that make natural carbohydrates so fattening. For example, one cup of potatoes is only 130 calories. Put one tablespoon of oil on top, and you just added another 100 calories!

Fat, such as olive oil, can be stored on your body within minutes, it is just packed away on your hips and waist. Foods cooked in oil or coated with oils soak up more fat than you think. A low-calorie "healthy food" quickly becomes fattening. If you are thin and exercise a lot, one or two tablespoons of oil a day is no big deal, but if you're trying to lose weight, the best choice is no oil at all.

Watching Blood Pressure?
Reduce Salt

We need sodium in our diet to be alive, but we need very little of it. Sodium is an important mineral that is essential to the body's proper function—however, adding salt (sodium chloride) to food provides us with dangerously high amounts of sodium.

Since salt is an ingredient in just about every type of processed food or restaurant meal, most people are getting double—or triple—the amount of sodium they need each day. Only 8 ounces of canned tomato soup can have as much as 1,200 milligrams of sodium. But high salt use is by no means limited to processed foods or fast-food restaurants. Even chefs of fine restaurants use excess salt. Since we already eat a lot of salt and are conditioned to high-salt taste, they find they must raise the salt levels in their food to stand out.

"For optimal health, I recommend that no salt at all be added to any food," says Dr. Joel Fuhrman, MD, in his book "Eat To Live," recommends that for optimal health no salt be added to any food.

The recipes in this book include salt, because I use it in small amounts, but ultimately it's your choice. Do what is right for you.

Making the Switch to Low Sodium Cooking

Human taste buds are highly adaptable little organs. If yours demand salty foods, you can reprogram them by cutting back gradually. The taste buds aren't sensitive enough to notice a reduction in the salt of about 10 percent—and in many foods, up to 25 percent.

As you cut back on salt, add in lemon, pepper, vinegar, fresh herbs and spices, and other sodium-free flavorings, or use a salt substitute as a bridge. Your taste buds will be happy without the need to settle for bland-tasting food. Over time, you might rediscover the real flavor of food and the complex tastes that herbs and spices have to offer. It will take 2-3 months for your senses to stop craving salt as much. The good news is that within three weeks, you should be able to discern a real difference in the taste of food and find the addition of salt unpleasant.

The Environmental Footprint of Foods

Many people, when they learn that I'm vegan, ask me about certain foods, like avocados, almonds, bananas, or soy, which they've heard were problematic for the environment. Avocados and almonds are said to use excessive amounts of water to grow, a fact that is widely discussed in the media lately.

Because many recipes in this book use avocados, and some may use almonds, the question is: What is the environmental impact of these foods? How bad are they compared to other foods?

And, finally, are avocados worse for the environment than beef? This issue is important to me, as it should be to all of us.

Whichever way you look at it, avocados are still a LOT better for the environment than animal products. An avocado in your raw soup, on a toast, or a small bowl of guacamole produces only a fraction of the greenhouse gas emissions and water used to produce the same amount of meat or cheese. Even so, you don't have to use avocados if you find them too problematic, too difficult to find, too expensive, or for any other reason. The updated version of this book provides a great alternative to emulsifying soups without avocados that is only slightly more time-consuming, but make up for it by producing a full-bodied raw soup that is based on a traditional favorite. (This version contains some oil, so it's a little higher in calories, something to be mindful of, if you are trying to lose weight.)

Another argument people use against eating a healthy plant-based diet is that it's too expensive. But it doesn't have to be! Try to buy locally grown ingredients that are in season, and reduce the waste as much as possible, to minimize the adverse impact. Grow your own fruits and veggies in your backyard. Planting a fruit tree is not time-consuming at all, and you'll get a nice crop of fresh produce every year! Buy from local farmers who use organic methods to grow their crops to support them. These products are usually the cheapest. And take your own shopping bags with you to avoid plastic waste.

Another thing to keep in mind is that meat production is heavily subsidized to make it cheaper for the consumer. Even vegans pay (through our taxes) for beef production, which is really frustrating. I would much rather see my tax dollars go to farmers growing fruits and vegetables, which are much better for our health and the environment. If the price of these products were to reflect the REAL cost of producing them, the price of meat and other animal products would be prohibitive.

Why Go Plant-Based?

The recipes in this book are entirely plant-based, and my reasons for including only vegan recipes go far beyond simple replacement of one product with another for the purpose of improving one's health, energy levels, and vitality (although that will happen too).

Now, I realize you are reading this book because you want to learn how to make delicious and healthy soups, and you may not be interested in being preached about the moral virtues of eating a plant-based diet.

I hear you.

I used to think that way too. After all, people have been consuming animal products for thousands of years! Few people ever bother to dig deeper, to find out more about the animals—how they live and how they die—and about the effects that eating animals has on our planet.

Perhaps the main reason for our avoidance of this topic is this. Once you learn the truth about animal exploitation, it's hard to go back. It's hard to keep eating things we are so used to and love as if nothing has happened.

When you think about it, it's mind-boggling that 65 billion land animals suffer and die every year so that we can enjoy the taste of their flesh and secretions. We never see them or know anything about the way they live and die. We never question the ethics behind it. Perhaps it's too painful to face the reality of what is happening behind the doors of animal farms and slaughterhouses. Maybe it's too inconvenient to have to switch to a totally new way of eating and living. Who has the time and energy to do that?

Like most people, I thought I could never go vegan because it was just too tough, too inconvenient, and… well… isolating. I didn't believe I could stick to it long term because I would feel too hungry, deprived, and just too different. Sort of like a "vegan freak."

Once I moved from ignorance to awareness, I realized it's really not that hard. Yes, it's inconvenient at times. Yes, some people will find it difficult to accept your new way of eating. However, I am now grateful to experience the bliss of total compassion and to live in such a way that celebrates all living beings.

So if you are skeptical or even annoyed that I even bring up this subject, I understand. Ultimately, it's your decision how you continue to live your life.

However, I encourage you to start by increasing your knowledge about the issue of raising animals for food. Learning to prepare these delicious soups will make it easier for you to take the first step towards reducing pain and suffering on this planet. Why not spread the love and compassion onto all living beings—by simply preparing tasty dishes that are also good for you.

3 Reasons to Choose Plant-Based & Vegan Diet & Lifestyle!

I can think of plenty of reasons to stop eating animal products. Here are the three most common:

1. Do It for the Animals

I list if as the first reason, because this is what finally convinced me to quit eating animal products altogether.

Once I mustered the courage to watch the video footage and read about what really happens to farmed animals, laboratory animals, as well as other animals that are exploited by humans, there was no turning back for me. I already knew that from the health perspective, there is no reason for humans to continue eating animal products. I knew what I had to do, and making the change has been easy.

If you are like me, you probably don't want to hear about the horrific treatment of animals that are raised for food, even before they are slaughtered. Like it or not, an enormous amount of suffering is involved, and by cutting out meat, you'll be reducing your involvement in that.

Ninety-nine percent of all land animals used for meat, milk, or eggs are factory farmed. Around 450 billion animals are factory farmed on our planet every year. What animals have to go through in these facilities is horrific.

The treatment of dairy cows in factory farms is probably the worst. We often forget (or prefer not to think about) the simple fact that cows, like other mammals, only produce milk after giving birth. They don't just "give milk"; cows are repeatedly and forcefully inseminated and kept pregnant over much of their lifetime, while their babies (calves), considered a mere byproduct of the process, are killed (that's where veal comes from).

Chickens are now specifically bred for either eating or laying eggs. Male "egg-laying" chicks, unable to fulfill their purpose, are killed right away, often very inhumanely.

The over-fishing of our oceans has led to a dangerously dramatic decline in wildlife. For every ten tuna, shark, and other large predatory fish in our oceans fifty to a hundred years ago, only one is left. Many species are on the verge of extinction for being "accidentally" killed because of modern fishing practices. For every one pound of shrimp, approximately twenty-six pounds of other sea animals are killed and tossed back into the ocean.

The over-fishing of our oceans has led to a dangerously dramatic decline in wildlife. For every ten tuna, shark, and other large predatory fish in our oceans fifty to a hundred years ago, only one is left. Many species are on the verge of extinction for being "accidentally" killed because of modern fishing practices. For every one pound of shrimp, approximately twenty-six pounds of other sea animals are killed and tossed back into the ocean.

2. Do It for the Planet

Animal farming is the number one cause of climate change in the world. In fact, it has a 40% larger carbon footprint than all transportation around the globe combined. This means that every car, truck, bus, train, and plane combined are almost half as bad for our planet as modern animal farming.

Animal farming is a massive drain on resources like water and grain. It takes 2,500 gallons of water to produce a pound of meat, compared to only 25 gallons to produce a pound of grain. 70% of the grain grown in the US is used for producing meat. Currently, a third of the land on our planet is used to raise farm animals. If all that grain were being fed directly to people, no one would have to go hungry.

3. Do It for Yourself

Few of us question the morality of eating animals, and even people who feel its absolutely wrong do it anyway out of habit. **Eating with a clear conscience—feeling good about everything you put in your mouth—lightens up your life.** This goes beyond simple substitution, one ingredient for another in the name of better health or decreased waistline, even though that will happen too.

Scientific studies supported by the American Dietetic Association have confirmed that the vegan diet is associated with lower cholesterol, lower risk of heart disease, lower blood pressure, lower risk of hypertension and Type 2 diabetes, lower body fat, and lower overall cancer rates. In fact, studies have shown that a vegan diet can actually reverse diabetes, heart disease, and even cancer. The vegan diet is low in saturated fat and cholesterol, have higher levels of dietary fiber, magnesium and potassium, vitamins C and E, and folate.

The health benefits of a vegan lifestyle are vast. The American Dietetic Association (or ADA) released a report which stated that vegans "meet and exceed requirements" for protein consumption. In fact, vegans who consume whole nutrient-dense plant foods usually have better protein consumption than people who eat meat, dairy, and eggs.

Join the Revolution!

By becoming vegan, you are being the change that the world so desperately needs.

By becoming vegan, you are standing on the side of those who are helpless, who are invisible, who have no power, no voice.

By becoming vegan, you are the trend-setter. You are at the forefront of the REVOLUTION.

You are helping billions who cannot defend themselves.

You are the proof that one can live in accordance with one's values of compassion and justice; that your convenience or culinary pleasure is not a reason enough to inflict pain and to kill.

You are helping to set new standards—beyond just restaurant menus and what's served on your table every day.

It's not about broccoli or cashews or carrots—it's a revolution of consciousness, ethics, and values.

It's bigger than anything you ever witnessed before.

It's the next step in human development and the history of the world as we know it.

It's not a diet; it's a lifestyle and social justice movement.

It's a social justice fight that you're joining armed with a spoon and a fork.

Ending the biggest oppression, stopping the biggest crime committed by humans in the history of our civilization.

It can happen with or without you. It's a choice that everybody makes every single day.

When this happens, you'll be able to look back and say—I did that.

When your children or grandchildren ask you where you were when that change was happening, and what you did for the animals to end that holocaust—you'll be proud of yourself that you helped that movement grow. That you were not on the wrong side of history and justice. That you did the right thing.

Even if you hate broccoli. Or tofu. Or carrots.

I'm not crazy about broccoli myself. (You can always blend broccoli into a green smoothie. And carrots are delicious! Just try them in your JUICE!)

But you know what matters.

And you are ready to make the right choices. To take responsibility for your actions. And start being the human being that you always believed you were.

The Revolution Starts in Your Kitchen

By using the recipes in this book and taking the next step and becoming vegan (if you choose so, and I really hope you do!), you will be committing small acts of kindness every day—to your body, to the planet, and the animals. You'll be saying:

Hell-NO! to cruelty and violence.

NO! to exploiting mothers and their babies.

NO! to taking something that doesn't belong to you.

NO! to cave dweller mentality—we left the caves long ago, so why are we still behaving as if we belong there?

NO! to using (and abusing) someone for your pleasure and gain.

Now, I don't want anybody to think that I'm a negative, bitter, and angry person, and we don't want people to think about you either.

So here is the same thing stated in a positive way ;-).

By eating vegan, you'll be saying:

YES! to optimal health and wellness.

YES! to taking good care of your body.

YES! to compassion and living your deepest values.

YES! to caring about others, regardless of their race or species.

YES! to being gentle and caring.

YES! to evolving to the next stage of development of the human spirit and mind.

YES! to re-inventing traditions and customs and creating new ones—that suit our evolved consciousness.

YES! to justice for all.

YES! to peace and love.

And if you think that this is some kind of vegan propaganda, that I'm imposing my views on you and that everyone should be able to make their own choices with regards to food—then I ask you to watch some videos of what happens to animals who are raised for food. Read some books. Watch some movies. Then ask yourself if that's okay with you. Whether you can, with clear conscience, condone that. And know that if the answer is 'No' then there is only one choice, and by now, I'm sure you know what to do.

Small Acts of Kindness Every Day— In Your Kitchen

What you do every day matters.

Your small every-day choices, compounded over time, make a difference. So, what is it going to be?

Thank You!

Thank you for reading!

I hope you feel inspired to start taking action.

If you enjoyed this book, I would appreciate a kind review on the booksellers' page.

Recommended Books

Many physicians recommend the whole plant food diet. If you want more information from a licensed physician, I recommend books by Dr. Joel Fuhrman, T.C. Campbell, Dr. Esselstyn, Dr. Neal Barnard, and others who promote this lifestyle.

Podcasts

Listen to them when you chop your veggies for soups and salads, when you exercise, drive to work or walk your dog.

Food For Thought (https://www.colleenpatrickgoudreau.com/podcast/) podcast by Colleen Patrick-Goudreau

It's All About Food (https://responsibleeatingandliving.com/its-all-about-food-2/) by Caryn Hartglass.

Bonus Excerpt from the "Easy Green Smoothie Recipe Book for Kids & Adults: Get Your Family Drinking Greens, Fruits & Veggies with Green Reset Formula!"

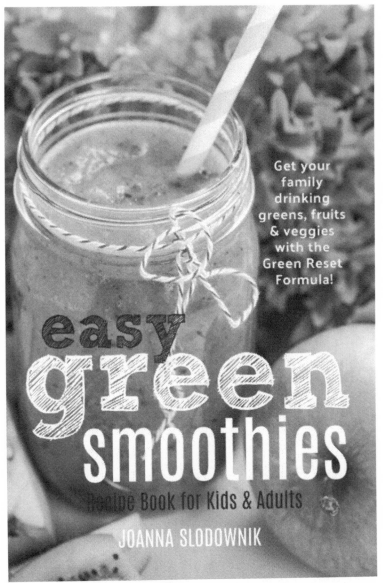

Rich & Creamy Smoothie Recipes

Banana Almond Butter Smoothie

    1 ½ cup almond milk, or any other dairy-free milk

    2-3 cups mild greens, such as spinach or mixed greens

    3 bananas
    1 cup peaches or other fruit, fresh or frozen
    2 tablespoons almond butter (or nut butter of your choice)
    ½ teaspoon vanilla butter or extract
    Yields about 1.5 quart

Cinnamon Banana Blast Smoothie

    1 ½ cup water (or more for a thinner smoothie)
    2-4 cups baby spinach or kale
    ½ cup any type of cooked whole grain
    1 ripe banana
    ½ teaspoon cinnamon
    1 tablespoon walnuts
    Yields about 1 quart

Mixed Berry Blast Smoothie

    2 cups water or non-dairy milk (or more for a thinner smoothie)
    2-4 cups greens (kale, collards, parsley, or other)
    2-3 stalks of celery
    ¼ small avocado
    1 cup mixed berries, frozen
    1 apple, cored and chopped
    1 banana
    1 cup cooked grains
    Yields about 2 quarts

Avocado Vanilla Smoothie

    1 cup almond milk ½ avocado
    2 chopped, pitted dates
    2 teaspoons vanilla extract
    2 teaspoons agave nectar
    Yields about a half quart

Spicy Plum Oat Smoothie

2 cups non-dairy milk (or more for a thinner smoothie)
1-2 cups spinach
8 plums
1 banana
1 cup oats, cooked quinoa, or brown rice
½ cup dates
½ teaspoon vanilla
1 teaspoon fresh ginger
Yields about 1.5 quarts

Peachy Green Smoothie

1 cup non-dairy milk (or more for a thinner smoothie)
1 cup spinach
3 small peaches, pitted
1 tablespoon sesame seeds
¼ cup dried apricots (pre-soaked for a smoother blend)
½ cup instant oats
sprinkle with a dash of cinnamon before serving
Yields about 1 quart

Strawberry Oat Smoothie

1 cup oat milk or other non-dairy milk
1 cup water, or to desired consistency
1 cup strawberries
2 cups spinach
2 large stalks of celery
1 banana
1 cup instant oats
2 tablespoons pumpkin seeds Yields about 2 quarts

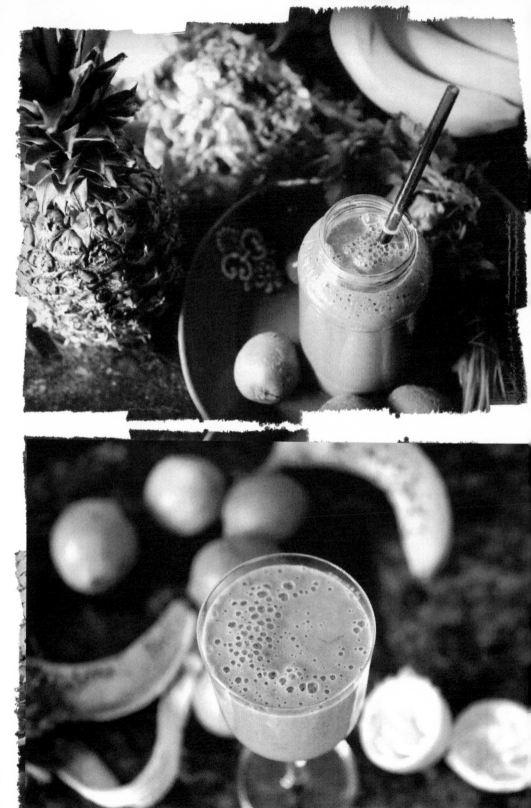

Healthy & Decadent Dessert Recipes

When making blended desserts, I usually don't include greens in them, so technically, they don't belong in this book. However, I wanted to include a few recipes, at least to get you started with some simple combinations. My three favorite base ingredients are frozen bananas, avocado, tofu, and chia seeds.

Although adding greens or vegetables to a dessert may seem wicked, if you don't overdo it, your child will not even notice.

I would stick to avocado or celery to avoid changing the color.

Preparing the dessert with frozen fruit or adding some ice will make the taste of greens even less noticeable.

Banana Almond Dessert

2 very ripe bananas, frozen
2 tablespoons almond butter
½ celery stalk
2 chopped, pitted dates
1 cup water or almond milk
Combine all ingredients and blend until very smooth.

Frozen Mango Banana Smoothie

3 medium frozen bananas or more, depending on desired thickness
1 mango
¼ medium avocado
2 teaspoons maple syrup or agave nectar
1 cup water or almond milk
Add frozen bananas and blend until smooth. Enjoy immediately!

Easiest Ever Chocolate Mousse

1 large avocado (3/4—1 cup mashed)
1/4 —1/3 cup vegan hot cocoa mix (sweetened)
a pinch of salt
a few drops of vanilla extract
Mash up the avocado with hot cocoa mix. Process in a food processor until smooth with a pinch of salt and a few drops of vanilla. Serve in pretty glass containers decorated with slices of banana, chocolate chips, coconut flakes, or whatever else you have in your pantry!

Read More Books:
The Green Reset Formula

Get more **Green Reset Formula Books with 100+ Easy Recipes for Healthy Living**, including:

Green Reset! 6-Week Green Smoothie and Juicing Challenge (with recipes, shopping lists, tips, detox advice, and more)

Easy Green Smoothie Recipe Book for Kids & Adults: Get Your Family Drinking Greens, Fruits & Veggies

Easy Soups! Creamy, Thick & Satisfying Soups That Will Fill You Up

Your Gift Is Waiting!

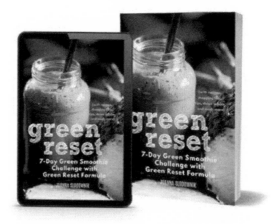

To get the free "7-Day Green Smoothie Challenge" go to JoannaSlodownik.com/gift/

Made in the USA
Las Vegas, NV
18 October 2022

57624547R00046